THE DIABETES RECIPES

COOKBOOK FOR BEGINNERS

A Complete Guide to Manage Diabetes Symptoms with Low-Sugar Dishes

TABLE OF CONTENT

INTRODUCTION____________________________________5

CHAPTER ONE____________________________________8

HOW DIABETES DEVELOPS IN THE BODY__8
TYPE 1 DIABETES _____________________9
TYPE 2 DIABETES _____________________13
GESTATIONAL DIABETES _____________15

CHAPTER TWO___________________________________19

CARBOHYDRATE COUNTING_______________19
Right Amount of Carbs to Eat ____20

GLYCEMIC INDEX_________________________22
What you need to know ___________23
Benefits of Low GI Foods For
Diabetes _________________________________25

CHAPTER THREE_________________________________27

LOW-SUGAR & LOW-CARB RECIPES ______27
Homemade Buttermilk Pumpkin
Waffles _________________________________27
Mini Quiche ____________________________30
Sausage and Brussels Sprouts
Scrambled Eggs ________________________32
Breakfast Quinoa Bowl with
Blackberries ____________________________35

English Muffin Breakfast Sandwich _________________________________37
Banana Pancakes _____________________38
Potato Cauliflower Scramble _____41
Mango & coconut muffins _________44
Roasted Carrot Quinoa Salad _____46
Green Bean, Walnut, and Feta Salad _________________________________49
Apple Pecan Arugula Salad _______51
Sweet & Crunchy Carrot Salad ____53
Chicken Caesar Salad ____________55
Spinach Salad with Salmon _______58
Orange and Blueberry Fruit Salad 59
Peach Raspberry Smoothie ________61
Strawberries and Cream Smoothie _62
Silky Smoothie __________________63
Red Velvet Smoothie _____________64
Banana Chai Smoothie ____________65
CONCLUSION_______________________67

INTRODUCTION

Diabetes is a lifelong disease that can affect both children and adults. This disease is the sixth leading cause of death in the United States. It claims about 178,000 lives each year. Type one diabetes, also known as insulin dependent diabetes mellitus, usually occurs in people less than thirty years of age, but it also may appear at any age. Diabetes is a very serious disease with many life-threatening consequences, but if it is taken care of properly, diabetics can live a normal life.

Many of these problems can be prevented by having a low fat, low alcohol diet, maintaining a reasonable body mass, and working out thirty minutes five days a week. Performing these activities can also help reduce the risk of getting diabetes. There are many risk factors that one should take into consideration.

Having high blood pressure, being inactive and overweight are both very high-risk factors.

If a family member has diabetes or if a person is African, American Indian, Asian, Pacific Islander, Hispanic or Latino descent, they also have a greater risk of the disease.

Diet is the most important part of diabetes management. Without a proper diet, the amount of drugs and insulin needed to control blood sugar levels may be inadequate. Diet control helps reduce high blood sugar and reduce the risk of complications like heart attacks and high blood pressure. It also helps achieve ideal body weight and reduces the problems associated with obesity.

Diabetes can also lead to other health conditions, including kidney failure, eye disease, foot ulceration and a higher risk of heart disease. In our body we have a gland called the pancreas, inside the pancreas there are small beta cells, and these are the cells that produce chemicals called insulin for our body.

When we eat carbohydrate foods, the food are broken down into glucose, the glucose then travels to the bloodstream so that it can be used as energy for the different cells around the body.

CHAPTER ONE

HOW DIABETES DEVELOPS IN THE BODY

Diabetes is a complicated condition which can take many different forms. In addition to the more common types of diabetes which are; type 1, type 2 and gestational diabetes, there are other range of other types of diabetes, which are just as important. And about 2% of people have these other types of diabetes. These include different types of monogenic diabetes, cystic fibrosis-related diabetes, and diabetes caused by rare syndromes.

Certain medications such as steroids and antipsychotics could lead to other types of diabetes, as well as surgery or hormonal imbalances. Unfortunately, I have seen that many of the people have encountered are mostly misdiagnosed leading to delays in getting the right treatment.

To ensure better diagnosis and treatments for your type of diabetes, this chapter will teach you a lot about different diabetic conditions.

TYPE 1 DIABETES

If you have type 1 diabetes, your blood sugar is too high because your body can't make a hormone called insulin. There is nothing you can do to prevent yourself or others developing type 1 diabetes because the exact causes are not known. Although it's often diagnosed in childhood, but type 1 diabetes can develop at any age. You are at a slightly higher risk of type 1 diabetes if your mother, father, brother or sister has it.

Insulin is the main treatment for type 1 diabetes. You can't live without insulin injections or using an insulin pump. Checking and managing your blood sugar levels is important to help you reduce your risk of serious short or long-term health problems. These are called diabetes complications.

Symptoms

- Going for a wee more often, especially at night.

- Being constantly thirsty and not being able to quench it.

- Being incredibly tired and having no energy.

- Losing weight without trying to, or looking thinner than usual.

Know that we are not the same. You may also experience other symptoms and the symptoms you may have might not exactly match those of another person. If type 1 diabetes is left undiagnosed, it can make you really ill, really quickly. It can lead to a condition called diabetic ketoacidosis (DKA) which you can die from so please be cautious!

The symptoms of type 1 diabetes tend to come on quickly over just a few days or weeks. This is especially true in children. That's why it's important to see a doctor as soon as possible if you notice any of the signs. And it's important to know that type 1 diabetes and the symptoms you have won't exactly match those of another person.

Treatments

- Insulin is the main treatment for type 1 diabetes. If you have type 1 diabetes, your body doesn't make any insulin like it normally would. And you can't live without insulin as it helps you manage your blood sugar levels and prevent serious short or long-term health problems known as diabetes complications. So you'll need daily insulin injections or use an insulin pump a small device that you attach to your body which releases insulin. Your body will respond better to the insulin if you're healthy and active and it could help prevent insulin resistance which makes it harder to manage your blood sugar levels.

- Learning how to carb count helps you manage your blood sugar levels. It means you can match how much insulin you need for the carbohydrate you eat and drink. The sums can be made quicker and easier if you use certain apps or an insulin pump or closed loop system as many of the calculations are done for you.

- If you have type 1 diabetes you need to check your blood sugar levels regularly usually with a finger prick test. Being able to monitor your sugar levels without doing so many finger prick checks is made possible by using a CGM or flash glucose monitor. It also means you can spot and treat low and high blood sugar levels (hypos and hypers) more quickly. Some people with type 1 diabetes may also use a closed-loop system, also called an artificial pancreas. It's another way to help you manage your type 1 diabetes without having to do much of the work yourself.

Others ways to help you manage your type 1 diabetes and blood sugar levels include:

- Being as physically active as you can be

- Maintaining a healthy weight

- Going on a diabetes education course to get tips and information

- Going to your healthcare appointments and make sure you get your diabetes checks

TYPE 2 DIABETES

Type 2 diabetes is the most common type. It is high blood sugar levels due to your body not making enough of a hormone called insulin, or what it makes not working properly known as insulin resistance.

Type 2 diabetes can go undiagnosed for years if symptoms are missed. Left untreated high blood sugar levels can cause serious health problems called diabetes complications. Anyone can develop type 2 diabetes but it mostly affects people over 25 often with a family history. Type 2 diabetes doesn't just affect people living with overweight or obesity, although this is one of the risk factors, along with ethnicity. And there's no cure but with type 2 diabetes you can put your diabetes into remission by losing a significant amount of weight.

Symptoms

A lot of people don't get any signs or symptoms of type 2 diabetes or don't notice them. Symptoms can include:

- Weeing a lot, especially at night.

- Being really thirsty.

- Feeling more tired than usual.

- Losing weight without trying to and getting thinner.

- Genital itching or thrush.

- Cuts and wounds taking longer to heal.

- Blurred eyesight.

Treatments

The main treatments for managing blood sugar levels if you have type 2 diabetes are:

- Eating well and moving more

- Weight loss

- Metformin (usually taken as a tablet)

- Insulin along with other medication that helps lower blood sugar levels

- Other types of diabetes medicine that is injected or taken as tablets.

- Weight loss surgery

GESTATIONAL DIABETES

Gestational diabetes is diabetes that can develop during pregnancy. It affects women who haven't been affected by diabetes before. It means you have high blood sugar and need to take extra care of yourself and your bump. This will include eating well and keeping active.

It usually goes away again after giving birth. It is usually diagnosed from a blood test 24 to 28 weeks into pregnancy. If you've found out you have gestational diabetes, you're not alone.

You'll get lots of extra care and support from your care team at every stage

Symptoms

Gestational diabetes is a type of diabetes that develops during pregnancy. It affects women who haven't already got a diagnosis of another type of diabetes. It means you have high blood sugar and need to take extra care of yourself and your bump. This will include eating well and keeping active. It usually goes away again after giving birth.

Signs and symptoms associated with gestational diabetes include:

- Going for a wee a lot, especially at night.

- Being really thirsty.

- Feeling more tired than usual.

- Genital itching or thrush.

- Blurred eyesight.

You may have been shocked to find out that you have gestational diabetes, many women have no noticeable symptoms. As some gestational diabetes symptoms are like symptoms experienced in pregnancy anyway like feeling more tired or going to the toilet more. Most cases are diagnosed during screening for gestational diabetes. This is called an Oral Glucose Tolerance Test, also known as an OGTT.

The OGTT is usually done when you're between 24-28 weeks pregnant. If you've had gestational diabetes before, you'll be offered the OGTT or self-monitoring of your blood sugar levels at home early in your pregnancy. You'll be shown how to do this and given a blood monitoring kit.

CHAPTER TWO

CARBOHYDRATE COUNTING

Diabetes is a chronic health condition that occurs when too much sugar, or glucose, is in the blood. Fortunately, with proper treatment and dietary changes, adverse health outcomes can be prevented. One diabetes meal planning technique that is used to manage blood glucose is carb counting, which is slightly different from calorie counting. Carb counting involves keeping track of the carbs in your snacks, meals, and beverages to manage blood sugar levels.

The carbohydrates in foods we eat break down into glucose, which causes your blood sugar to rise. Normally, when blood glucose goes up, the pancreas releases insulin. Insulin is a hormone made in the pancreas that enables blood glucose in the body's cells to be used for energy. For people with diabetes, the body is unable to use insulin properly or produce enough insulin. This leads to high glucose levels circulating in the blood.

Why Should you Count Carbs? Carb counting is a flexible way to eat the foods you enjoy while maintaining a low-carb diet. It also helps you learn how certain foods affect your blood sugar so you can match the foods you eat to your insulin dose.

Right Amount of Carbs to Eat

As an adult with diabetes, you should aim to get 45–60 grams of carbs per meal and 15–30 grams of carbs per snack. For diabetes meal planning, one carb serving is equal to 15 grams of carbohydrates.

Here are some foods that have around 15 grams of carbohydrates:

- 1 slice bread

- ⅓ cup of pasta or rice

- 2 rice cakes

- ½ cup of oatmeal

- 1 cup of low-fat milk

- ⅔ cup of light yogurt

- ½ cup of fruit juice

- ½ cup of beans

- 3 cups of raw vegetables

- half of a potato or a similar portion of other starchy vegetables

- Non-starchy vegetables, including carrots, asparagus, and leafy greens like broccoli and spinach, are much lower in carbohydrates than starchy vegetables. For instance, one-half cup of cooked broccoli contains just 5 grams of carbohydrates.

- Protein and fat sources do not contain enough carbohydrates to count toward your daily allowance. However, they are important to include in each meal to slow the uptake of glucose in your bloodstream and provide you with energy.

GLYCEMIC INDEX

Living with diabetes can be mentally hard to deal with for some people. However, it need not be something to fear. Diabetes, although chronic, can be effectively managed with little tweaks in our lifestyle and diet. But how do we know exactly what we should eat to manage our diabetes? Some might say cut out sugar entirely, others cut out carbohydrates entirely, some might even subject you to bland food all your life now that you're diabetic. However, many diabetics have gone on to live happy and healthy lives without compromising on the taste of their foods.

Substituting your favorite foods with simple healthy swaps can help you manage your blood sugar as well as help your taste buds adapt to a palette that will benefit you in the long run. Doctors recommend diabetics should include foods that have a low glycemic index. Having a glycemic index chart in place can help you choose what foods to include and what to limit in or eat in limited portions in your diabetic diet.

Understanding the glycemic index of foods helps you assess how much each food affects your blood sugar levels. Once you have that knowledge, it is easier to plan your meal accordingly.

The glycemic index not only helps you be aware of what you are putting in your body but also helps in maintaining your weight loss journey and keeping your cholesterol in check. So let us take a detailed look into what glycemic index is, how it affects our diet and how it helps us control our sugar levels?

What you need to know

The Glycemic Index is a rating tool or a measuring system that gives you an idea about how much a particular food can increase your blood sugar levels. It is used to promote healthy eating habits and help diabetic patients increase awareness of what to eat in order to keep their weight, cholesterol and blood sugar levels under control.

The glycemic index of a food is determined based on various factors such as nutritive composition, ripeness of the food, how processed it is, sugar content and its cooking time and method. Foods are generally rated from 0 – 100 and are called low, medium or high glycemic food based on their ratings.

The three glycemic index ratings are:

- Low glycemic foods – 55 or below

- Medium glycemic foods – 56 – 69

- High glycemic foods – 70 or above

For better understanding, the lower the glycemic rating, the longer the food takes to digest, bringing a slower rise in your blood sugar levels.

Foods with a high glycemic index are usually digested quickly which makes you hungry sooner. If you eat more high glycemic foods, you will end up eating more unhealthy foods which would result in weight gain and high blood sugar levels.

While the Glycemic index is used to determine how much a particular food increases your blood sugar levels, it does not reflect on the quantity of the food.

For this purpose, researchers came up with the idea of a Glycemic load. A Glycemic Load shows the number of calories you will be consuming, in a serving of that particular food. This helps you determine how much to eat in a serving in order to maintain your blood sugars.

The three glycemic load ratings are:

- 10 or lower – Low Glycemic load

- 11 – 19 – Medium Glycemic load

- 20 or higher – High Glycemic load

Benefits of Low GI Foods For Diabetes

One of the most crucial ways to control diabetes is by monitoring your blood sugar levels. Only if you are mindful of what you eat and how much of it you eat, will you be able to control and maintain your weight, blood sugar levels and a number of other health complications that arise with diabetes. And ultimately, the only way to be mindful of your meals is by calculating the Glycemic index and load of each meal.

Foods with a low glycemic index often keep you full for a longer period of time since they take a longer time to digest. These foods are high in fibre and protein while high GI foods consist of hidden sugars and refined carbohydrates. Therefore, it is advisable for diabetic patients or any person who's trying to maintain their weight, to swap high GI food for low GI food.

Some benefits of swapping high GI foods for low GI foods are:

- Improved blood sugar regulation

- Speeds up weight loss

- Decreases cholesterol levels

- Improves Blood Pressure

CHAPTER THREE

LOW-SUGAR & LOW-CARB RECIPES

Homemade Buttermilk Pumpkin Waffles

Total Time: 30 Minutes

Ingredients

- 2 cups all-purpose flour

- 3/4 cup granulated sugar

- 3 teaspoons baking powder

- 1/4 teaspoon kosher salt

- 1 teaspoon ground cinnamon

- 1/4 teaspoon pumpkin pie spice

- 2 large eggs whites and yolks separated

- 1 cup buttermilk

- 1/2 cup milk I used 2%

- 1 cup unsalted butter melted

- 1 teaspoon pure vanilla extract

- 1/2 cup pumpkin puree

- 1 stick unsalted butter

- 1/2 cup granulated sugar

- 1/2 cup buttermilk

- 1/2 teaspoon baking soda

- 1/2 teaspoon pure vanilla extract

Directions

- Preheat waffle iron.

- Place flour, sugar, baking powder, salt, cinnamon and pumpkin pie spice into a large mixing bowl, stir to combine.

- Place egg whites into a medium mixing bowl, whisk continuously until stiff peaks form.

- Place buttermilk, milk, melted butter, vanilla and egg yolks into a large bowl, whisk to combine then slowly stir into dry ingredients. Stir in pumpkin puree then gently fold in egg whites until just combined.

- Scoop 1/2 cup of batter and place into center of waffle iron, close lid and let cook until golden brown and crisp, about 2 1/2 minutes depending on your waffle iron. Remove hot waffles and place on cooling rack. Continue cooking waffles until all batter is used.

- To prepare buttermilk syrup, place butter, sugar and buttermilk into a small saucepan. Stir until melted and comes to a low boil. Remove from heat and stir in baking soda and vanilla. Syrup will foam up. Let sit aside and stir occasionally until foam has gone down.

Mini Quiche

Total Time: 45 Minutes

Ingredients

- 5 eggs

- 1 cup milk or heavy cream

- ¾ tsp. salt

- ¼ tsp. black pepper

- ¼ tsp. garlic powder

- 2 pie crusts 14 oz. total

- ½ cup cheese cheddar or Swiss

- 1 cup add-ins bacon, mushrooms, bell peppers, chives, etc.

Directions

- Whisk together eggs, milk, salt, pepper, and garlic powder in a large bowl with a spout or in a large measuring cup. Refrigerate until ready to use.

- Roll out dough on a lightly floured cutting board until it is at least 12-inches round in diameter. Use a 2 ½-inch round cookie cutter to cut 24 circles from each sheet of pie crust. You will end up re-rolling the dough about 3-4 times.

- Press pie crust rounds into the bottoms of a mini muffin tray that has been sprayed liberally with non-stick cooking spray. Press up the sides so the crust completely covers them.

- Fill each pie crust with 1 teaspoon of add-ins and a sprinkle of cheese.

- Pour in egg mixture and fill up just shy of the top of the pie crust. Use a small spoon to mix together all of the add-ins and cheese so they're evenly distributed throughout the egg mixture.

- Bake at 375 for 20-22 minutes, or until the pie crust is golden and the egg middle no longer jiggles.

- Serve immediately with a sprinkle of fresh herbs and enjoy!

Sausage and Brussels Sprouts Scrambled Eggs

Total Time: 20 Minutes

Ingredients

- 8 large eggs

- 1 1/2 tbsp coconut milk, unsweetened canned

- 1 pack chicken apple sausages

- 2 cups Brussels sprouts, quartered

- 1/2 cup yellow onion slices

- 1 tbsp olive oil

- 1/2 tsp pink sea salt

- 1/2 tsp cracked pepper

- 1/4 tsp garlic powder

- 3 tsp ghee

Directions

- Clean and quarter the Brussels sprouts and slice the yellow onions. Remove the sausage from the package and slice as desired.

- Heat a medium size skillet over medium/high heat with 1 tbsp olive oil.

- First, add in the sausage along with the onions and cook for 5 minutes.

- Next, add the Brussels sprouts to the sausage and onion mixture along with 1 tsp pf ghee, garlic powder, 1/4 tsp salt and 1/4 tsp pepper.

Allow to cook until the Brussels sprouts become tender (I would say another 7 minutes).

- While the sausage mixture is cooking, heat up another skillet over medium heat along with 2 tsp of ghee. Add 8 large eggs to a medium size bowl along with 1 1/2 tbsp canned coconut milk and the remainder 1/4 tsp salt and 1/4 tsp pepper. Whisk/beat together until combined.

- Once skillet is hot, pour in the egg mixture. As the eggs begin to heat up, gently pull the egg mixture back and forth with a spatula until the egg mixture becomes firm. Fold the eggs until there is no liquid and the eggs are solid.

- Remove the eggs and add desired amount to plate and serve the sausage and Brussels sprout mixture over the top. ENJOY!

Breakfast Quinoa Bowl with Blackberries

Total Time: 30 Minutes

Ingredients

- 1 cup uncooked quinoa

- 1 cup unsweetened almond milk

- 1 cup water

- ½ teaspoon ground cinnamon

- 2 cups fresh or frozen blackberries

- 1/3 cup chopped pecans toasted

- 4 teaspoons maple syrup

Directions

- Place the uncooked quinoa in a dry medium pan (with no oil or butter), and cook over medium heat for about 5 to 7 minutes, stirring frequently, or until you hear a little popping,

and the quinoa will small nutty and toasty.
Keep an eye on the quinoa, and be careful not
to burn it!

- Pour the milk and water, and mix the
  cinnamon into the toasted quinoa, and
  continue to cook over medium heat. Bring to
  a boil, then reduce the heat to low, and cover
  and simmer 15 minutes or until most of the
  liquid is absorbed. Turn off heat, and let stand
  covered 5 minutes. Stir in blackberries.
  Transfer to four serving bowls and top with
  pecans. Drizzle 1 teaspoon maple syrup over
  each serving.

- While the quinoa cooks, roast the pecans in a
  350° F degree oven for 5 to 6 minutes. Or
  toast nuts in a dry skillet on the stovetop over
  medium heat for about 3 minutes. Or toast in
  an air fryer, by placing the nuts in the bottom
  of the basket in a single layer, you may use a
  piece of parchment paper to keep them from

falling through if you need to, set the cook temperature to 300° F, and air fry for 4-6 minutes.

English Muffin Breakfast Sandwich

Total Time: 20 Minutes

Ingredients

- 6 slices bacon cooked and crumbled

- 6 hard boiled eggs chopped

- 1 cup cheddar cheese

- ½ cup mayonnaise

- ½ tablespoon dijon mustard

- ¼ teaspoon garlic powder

- 1 teaspoon Worchestershire sauce

- 4 English muffins split muffins

Directions

- Preheat broiler.

- In a medium bowl, combine mayonnaise, mustard, garlic powder and Worcestershire sauce.

- Add chopped eggs and cheese and stir until just combined. Salt and pepper to taste.

- Open an English muffin and top with extra cheese and bacon pieces if desired. Place on the middle rack in the oven. Broil for 3-4 minutes, until cheese melts and muffins are slightly toasted. Watch carefully

Banana Pancakes

Total Time: 20 Minutes

Ingredients

- 1½ cups all purpose flour, spooned into measuring cup and leveled off

- 2 tablespoons sugar

- 2½ teaspoons baking powder

- ½ teaspoon salt

- 1 small, over-ripe banana, peeled (the browner, the better)

- 2 large eggs

- 1 cup plus 2 tablespoons low fat milk

- ½ teaspoon vanilla extract

- 3 tablespoons unsalted butter, melted

- 1 - 2 tablespoons vegetable oil

- 1 tablespoon unsalted butter

- Maple syrup

- Sliced bananas

- Confectioners' sugar (optional)

Directions

- In a medium bowl, whisk together the flour, sugar, baking powder and salt.

- In a small bowl, mash the banana with a fork until almost smooth. Whisk in the eggs, then add the milk and vanilla and whisk until well blended. Pour the banana mixture and the melted butter into the flour mixture. Fold the batter gently with a rubber spatula until just blended; do not over-mix. The batter will be thick and lumpy.

- Set a griddle or non-stick pan over medium heat until hot. Put a pad of butter and one tablespoon vegetable oil onto the griddle, and swirl it around. Drop the batter by ¼-cupfuls onto the griddle, spacing the pancakes about 2 inches apart. Cook until a few holes form on top of each pancake and the underside is golden brown, about 2 minutes. Flip the pancakes and cook until the bottom is golden brown and the top is puffed, 1 to 2 minutes more. Using the spatula, transfer the pancakes to a serving plate.

- Wipe the griddle clean with paper towels, add more butter and oil, and repeat with the remaining batter. Serve the pancakes while still hot with maple syrup, sliced bananas and confectioners' sugar if desired

Potato Cauliflower Scramble

Total Time: 20 Minutes

Ingredients

- 2-4 tablespoons water

- 1/2 cup chopped green onions or 3 tablespoons dried onion flakes

- 1 cup finely chopped zucchini

- 2 1/2 – 3 cups steamed cauliflower florets mashed

- 1 12–16-ounce package medium or medium-firm tofu, drained and crumbled

- 2 cups chopped cooked potato see note

- 1 teaspoon Dijon mustard

- 1/2 teaspoon garlic powder

- 1/4 teaspoon salt or more to taste

- Freshly ground black pepper to taste optional

- 2 tablespoons tahini

- 2 1/2 tablespoons nutritional yeast

- 1/2 – 3/4 teaspoon black salt see note

- 2-3 cups chopped spinach or kale optional

Directions

- Heat a large nonstick skillet over medium-high heat.

- Pour in 2 tablespoons water and add the onions and zucchini. Cook for 5 minutes, or until slightly softened, then add the cauliflower, tofu, potato, mustard, garlic powder, salt, and pepper (if desired).

- Cook for 3–4 minutes, then add the tahini and nutritional yeast and stir to combine. If the mixture is sticking to the pan, add another tablespoon or two of water.

- To finish, add the black salt; if you're using greens, add them and stir until just wilted and still bright green (spinach will cook faster than kale). Season to taste with extra salt, pepper, and black salt, and serve.

Total Time: 20 Minutes

Ingredients

- 2 cups wholemeal plain flour

- 2 teaspoons baking powder

- 1/2 cup brown sugar, plus extra to sprinkle

- 1 cup coconut, desiccated, plus extra to sprinkle

- ¾ cup (180ml) vegetable oil

- 2 eggs

- 1 cup thick natural yoghurt

- 1 teaspoon vanilla essence

- 1 large mango, diced

Directions

- Preheat oven to 180°C (350°F). Line a muffin tray with 12 muffin paper cases.

- Place flour, baking powder, brown sugar and coconut into a large bowl and mix to combine making a well in the centre. Place the oil, eggs, yoghurt and vanilla in a jug and whisk to combine. Pour the wet ingredients into the well of the dry and mix until just combined. Do not over mix. Add mango and gently fold to combine.

- Pour the mixture into the muffin cases (I use a ¼ cup measurement for this, super fast, clean and easy) and top each muffin with a sprinkling of brown sugar and coconut. Pop into the oven and bake for 15 – 20 minutes or until cooked (test by pressing gently on the top of the muffin, if the muffin bounces back they are done).

Roasted Carrot Quinoa Salad

Total Time: 45 Minutes

Ingredients

- 1 cup tricolor quinoa (or white, red or black quinoa)

- 2 cup water

- 1 ¼ pounds rainbow carrots

- 1 small red onion cut into ½-inch pieces

- 1 tablespoon olive oil

- 1 tablespoon pure maple syrup

- 2 teaspoons harissa

- ½ teaspoon garlic powder

- ½ teaspoon ground cumin

- ½ teaspoon kosher salt

- ¼ cup minced flat-leaf parsley

- 2 green onions thinly sliced

- ¼ cup fresh lemon juice

- 1 tablespoon plus 1 teaspoon pure maple syrup

- 1 garlic clove finely grated on a zester

- ¾ teaspoon ground cumin

- ½ teaspoon kosher salt

- ¼ teaspoon garlic powder

- ¼ teaspoon ground black pepper

Directions

- Place the quinoa in a fine mesh sieve and rinse well under running water. Transfer to a medium saucepan and add the water. Bring to a boil, then reduce heat to a simmer and cover.

Cook until the quinoa absorbs the water, 18 to 20 minutes.

- Fluff the quinoa with a fork. Transfer the quinoa to a large baking sheet and allow it to cool to room temperature. Transfer to a serving bowl.

- Preheat the oven to 425 degrees F.

- Cut the carrots into diagonal pieces about 1 inch long. As the carrots gets thicker, cut them in half lengthwise first. Pile the carrots and onions onto a large baking sheet.

- In a medium bowl, whisk together the olive oil, maple syrup, harissa, garlic powder, cumin and salt. Pour the mixture over the carrots and onions. Toss to coat.

- Roasted the vegetables until the carrots are tender, tossing them halfway through and transferring the baking sheet to the bottom rack of the oven to encourage further browning. Total cook time is 25-35 minutes, depending on the size of the carrots.

- After the vegetables cool for a few minutes, stir them into the quinoa, along with the parsley, green onion and dressing. Toss to combine. Serve.

- In a medium bowl, whisk together the lemon juice maple syrup, grated garlic, cumin, salt, garlic powder and pepper

Green Bean, Walnut, and Feta Salad

Total Time: 10 Minutes

Ingredients

- 2 pounds fresh green beans, trimmed

- 1 small purple onion, thinly sliced

- 1 (4-ounce) package crumbled feta cheese

- 1 cup coarsely chopped walnuts or pecans, toasted

- ¾ cup olive oil

- ¼ cup white wine vinegar

- 1 tablespoon chopped fresh dill

- ½ teaspoon minced garlic

- ¼ teaspoon salt

- ¼ teaspoon pepper

Directions

- Cut green beans into thirds, and arrange in a steamer basket over boiling water. Cover and steam 15 minutes or until crisp-tender. Immediately plunge into cold water to stop the cooking process; drain and pat dry.

- Toss together green beans, onion, cheese, and walnuts in a large bowl. Cover and chill 1 hour.

- Whisk together olive oil and next 5 ingredients; cover and chill 1 hour.

- Pour vinaigrette over green bean mixture, and chill 1 hour; toss just before serving.

Apple Pecan Arugula Salad

Total Time: 15 Minutes

Ingredients

- 1/2 cup raw pecans

- 7 ounces arugula (organic when possible)

- 2 small apples (1 tart, 1 sweet // peeled, quartered, cored and thinly sliced lengthwise)

- 1/4 red onion (thinly sliced)

- 2 Tbsp dried cranberries (optional)

- 1 large lemon, juiced (1 lemon yields ~3 Tbsp or 45 ml)

- 1 Tbsp maple syrup

- 1 pinch each sea salt plus black pepper

- 3 Tbsp olive oil

Directions

- Preheat oven to 350 degrees F (176 C) and arrange pecans on a bare baking sheet.

- Bake pecans for 8-10 minutes or until fragrant and deep golden brown. Remove from oven and set aside.

- While pecans are toasting, prep remaining salad ingredients and add to a large mixing bowl.

- Prepare dressing in a mixing bowl or mason jar by adding all ingredients and whisking or shaking vigorously to combine. Taste and adjust flavor as needed.

- Add pecans to salad and top with dressing. Toss to combine and serve immediately. Serves two as an entrée and 4 as a side.

- Store leftovers (dressing separate from salad) covered in the refrigerator for 2-3 days (though best when fresh). Dressing should keep at room temperature for 2-3 days when well-sealed.

Sweet & Crunchy Carrot Salad

Total Time: 20 Minutes

Ingredients

- 2 tablespoons extra-virgin olive oil

- 2 tablespoons freshly squeezed lemon juice

- 1 teaspoon spicy brown mustard

- 2 teaspoons pure maple syrup (or honey)

- 1/4 teaspoon fine sea salt

- freshly ground black pepper

- 1 pound carrots, peeled and shredded (about 4 heaping cups)

- 2 green onions, chopped (light green and white parts)

- 1 handful fresh parsley, chopped (about 1/4 cup packed)

- 1/2 cup raisins (optional)

- 1/2 cup pecans, roughly chopped (optional)

Directions

- In a large bowl, combine the olive oil, lemon juice, mustard, maple syrup, salt, and about 5 grinds of black pepper. Stir well.

- Add in the shredded carrots, green onions, and parsley, and gently toss everything together, to make sure the dressing coats all of the vegetables evenly. Taste and adjust the seasoning to your liking. You can add extra lemon juice if you want a more tart flavor, or a little more salt to punch up the flavor.

- Stir in the raisins and pecans, if using, and serve. If you don't plan on serving this salad right away, don't add the pecans because they will get softer in the fridge. Add the pecans right before serving if you make this in advance.

- Leftovers can be stored in an airtight container in the fridge for up to 3 days.

Chicken Caesar Salad

Total Time: 40 Minutes

Ingredients

- 4 chicken breasts

- 2 tablespoons olive oil divided

- 2 tablespoons cajun seasoning or to taste

- 8 cups romaine lettuce washed, dried

- 1 ½ cups croutons

- ¾ cup parmesan cheese grated

- 1 cup mayonnaise

- ¼ cup parmesan cheese grated

- 3 tablespoons lemon juice

- 1 tablespoon anchovy paste

- 2 teaspoons Worcestershire sauce

- 2 teaspoons dijon mustard

- 2 cloves garlic minced

Directions

- Combine all dressing ingredients and set aside.

- Combine the chicken breasts and 1 tablespoon olive oil in a small bowl. Season

with cajun spice, making sure to cover all of
the chicken.

- Heat up a large pan with remaining olive oil,
add the chicken once hot and cook on each
side ensuring that a dark crust is forming,
"blackening" the chicken.

- Cook until chicken has reached 165°F
internally or place in the oven to finish them.

- Once cooled, cut chicken breasts into slices.

- In a large bowl, cut romaine lettuce into bite
size pieces. Add croutons, parmesan cheese,
and prepared chicken. Top with dressing and
toss.

Spinach Salad with Salmon

Total Time: 15 Minutes

Ingredients

- 4 skinless salmon fillets (6 ounces each)

- coarse salt and pepper

- 10 ounces Baby Spinach

- 1 pint grape tomatoes, halved

- 3/4 cup crumbled fresh goat cheese (3 ounces)

- 1/4 cup pecans

- 1/4 cup balsamic-rosemary vinaigrette

Directions

- Heat broiler, with rack set 4 inches from heat. Place salmon on a foil-lined rimmed baking sheet; season with salt and pepper. Broil, without turning, until opaque throughout, 7 to 9 minutes. Let cool briefly, then flake.

- Divide spinach and tomatoes among serving plates. Top with salmon, goat cheese, and pecans, and drizzle with vinaigrette.

Orange and Blueberry Fruit Salad

Total Time: 30 Minutes

Ingredients

- 2 oranges (untreated)

- 1 lime (untreated)

- 1 dragon fruit

- 1 star fruit

- 7 ozs red grape

- 7 ozs white grape (seedless)

- 6 ozs raspberries

- 7 ozs strawberries

- 6 ozs blueberries

* 4 tbsps orange liqueur (or orange juice)

* 2 tbsps brown sugar

* mint (for garnish)

Directions

* Blanch oranges and lime in hot water, pat dry, quarter lengthwise and cut into slices.

* Peel dragon fruit and cut into pieces.

* Rinse and slice star fruit.

* Rinse grapes, cut in half and remove the seeds to taste.

* Rinse berries, remove stems and dice strawberries.

* Put everything in a bowl and mix with sugar and orange liqueur. Let rest about 10 min., then serve garnished with mint.

Peach Raspberry Smoothie

Total Time: 10 Minutes

Ingredients

- 1 cup sliced peaches

- 1/2 cup frozen raspberries

- 1 cup vanilla unsweetened almond milk or milk of your choice

- 1-2 teaspoons agave or honey depending on the sweetness of your peaches

- 3-4 ice cubes

Directions

- Add peaches and raspberries to blender

- Add milk, agave or honey, and ice cubes to the blender.

- Blend until smooth. Serve immediately.

Strawberries and Cream Smoothie

Total Time: 2 Minutes

Ingredients

- 1 1/4 cup frozen strawberries

- 3/4 cup almond milk

- 2 tablespoons fat-free half and half (may use almond milk instead)

- 1 tablespoon light brown sugar

- 1/4 teaspoon vanilla extract

Directions

- Place all ingredients into a blender.

- Pulse a few times to roughly chop the frozen strawberries before blending until drink is entirely smooth, about 1 minute.

- Serve immediately.

Total Time: 2 Minutes

Ingredients

- 1 can (354 mL) Fat Free Evaporated Skim Milk

- 1/2 cup (125 mL) orange juice

- 1 banana

- 1/3 cup (75 mL) Pure Strawberry Jam

- 1/2 cup (125 mL) frozen or fresh strawberries, sliced

- 2 tbsp (30 mL) Robin Hood Oats

Directions

- Combine all ingredients in blender. Blend until smooth. Thin with additional orange juice if desired. Enjoy immediately

Red Velvet Smoothie

Total Time: 5 Minutes

Ingredients

- 1 cup frozen mango, or 2 bananas

- 1 small beet (about 2 ounces), cooked and peeled. Start with 1/2 if you prefer

- 3 tablespoons cocoa powder

- 1.5 cup milk of choice, or to taste

- 3 dates, pitted

Directions

- Add all ingredients to your blender. Blend until smooth.

- Taste. Add more dates or mango for desired sweetness. Add more milk for desired consistency. Blend again and enjoy immediately.

Banana Chai Smoothie

Total Time: 5 Minutes

Ingredients

- 2 bananas, peeled, sliced and frozen

- 1 cup Blue Diamond Almond Breeze Almondmilk

- 1/2 cup plain non-fat Greek yogurt

- 2 teaspoons (dry) chai tea leaves

- 1 teaspoon vanilla extract, store-bought or homemade

- 1/4 teaspoon ground cinnamon

- (optional: 1 teaspoon maple syrup, if you'd like a sweeter smoothie)

Directions

- Add all ingredients to a blender and pulse until smooth.

Serve immediately, topped with a few extra slices of banana if desired.

CONCLUSION

In closing this cookbook crafted with care and consideration for those navigating the path of diabetes management, I want to extend my heartfelt gratitude for embarking on this culinary journey with me. Managing diabetes is a daily endeavor, and the choices we make in the kitchen play a crucial role in shaping our well-being.

As you savor the flavors of these diabetes-friendly recipes, remember that nourishing your body is a form of self-love. Each ingredient, each recipe, is a step toward a healthier and more vibrant life. Here are a few words of advice to carry with you on your ongoing culinary adventure:

Diversify your plate with a rainbow of colors and a spectrum of nutrients. Explore new ingredients and cooking techniques to keep your meals exciting and your body well-nourished.

Pay attention to portion sizes. Balancing your plate with the right proportions of carbohydrates, proteins, and healthy fats is key to managing blood sugar levels effectively.

Opt for whole grains, legumes, and vegetables as your primary sources of carbohydrates. These fiber-rich options have a gentler impact on blood sugar levels.

Include lean proteins in your meals to promote satiety and support muscle health. Fish, poultry, tofu, and legumes are excellent choices.

Choose sources of healthy fats, such as avocados, nuts, and olive oil. These fats contribute to overall well-being and help maintain stable blood sugar.

Stay well-hydrated with water, herbal teas, and other sugar-free beverages. Proper hydration is vital for overall health and can assist in managing blood sugar levels.

Establish a routine for your meals and snacks. Consistency in timing helps regulate blood sugar and promotes a stable energy supply throughout the day.

Work closely with your healthcare team to monitor your blood sugar levels regularly. Understanding your body's responses to different foods empowers you to make informed choices.

Cooking is a celebration of life and health. Approach it with joy and creativity. Experiment with flavors and discover the pleasure of crafting meals that both nourish and delight.

Everyone's body is unique. Pay attention to how different foods affect you personally. Your journey is individual, and adjustments may be needed to find what works best for you.

Remember, this cookbook is not just a collection of recipes but a companion in your daily quest for wellness.

As you savor the tastes, textures, and aromas of these dishes, let them be a source of inspiration, empowerment, and, above all, a delicious celebration of your commitment to a healthier, more flavorful life. Wishing you a journey filled with joy, vitality, and the satisfying embrace of good food on your path to wellness.